pulmonica®
Play More - Breathe Better

Pulmonica
HANDBOOK

Promotes deep belly breathing

Helps loosen congestion

No musical talent needed

Designed to always sound great

Breathe Better Now!

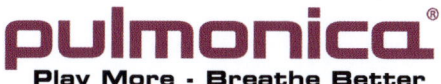

Play More - Breathe Better

Contents

About the Pulmonica® 3

The Pulmonica® Program 5

Pulmonica Care 14

Pulmonica Safety Information 16

Pulmonary Rehabilitation Therapy Basics 17

Pulmonary Rehabilitation Therapy Basics Continued 18

How do harmonicas work? 20

How is the Pulmonica different
from regular harmonicas? 21

What quality materials are used in
making the Pulmonica? 21

Who makes the Pulmonica? 22

How does Pulmonica differ from other respiratory therapy devices? 23

Why design a musical instrument for nonmusicians? 23

How was the Pulmonica developed? 23

Why are you giving so many away? 24

What type of research do you sponsor? 24

Do you sell in quantity? 24

I would like to play some simple songs, how can I learn? **24**

How long should the Pulmonica really last? **25**

I bought a Pulmonica for my family member, friend, neighbor, patient, etc. Is it all right to share? **26**

Something seems to be wrong with my Pulmonica. What should I do? **26**

For Medical Professionals **27**

Pulmonica® Research Results **28**

Testimonials included.. **31**

About the Pulmonica®

The Pulmonica is a specially constructed and tuned Pulmonary Harmonica® that produces deep, resonant, meditative sounds that can be felt vibrating in the lungs and sinuses. No musical talent is needed to use it – just breathing through the Pulmonica always sounds soothing. Smooth edges and quality materials make it safe to handle, easy to clean, and a joy to use.

The Pulmonica allows anyone to include conscientious belly breathing in their daily routine. Low harmonic frequencies gently pulse the lung and sinus cavities, helping to loosen secretions so they can be eliminated and make breathing easier. If breathing is a problem because of COPD, asthma, allergies, exposure to pollution, or other reasons, using the Pulmonica might help. Surveys and Amazon consumer reviews both show that the more people use one, the better they say they can breathe.

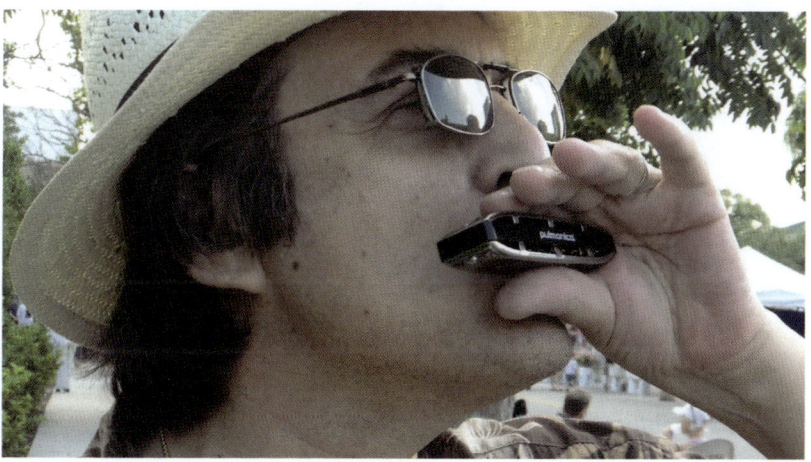

The special tuning makes the Pulmonica easy to use without a musical background. Wind instruments, especially harmonicas, have long been known to promote belly breathing (also referred to as abdominal or diaphragmatic breathing), but not everyone can learn to play a wind instrument. Long, slow, deep, and complete breathing is all that is needed to use a Pulmonica.

The primary markets for the Pulmonica are people with impaired lung function, including those with COPD, asthma, chronic bronchitis, cystic fibrosis. There are many conditions or situations where increased oxygenation and anxiety relief could be helpful including chronic fatigue, dementia, stress and mood disorders, wound healing, diabetes, post-surgical and trauma recovery in the general public and military, and smoking or other addiction cessation. Finally, the Pulmonica can help to increase diaphragmatic control and range of movement among musicians, athletes, stutterers, public speakers, obese people, and others who simply want to breathe better.

The Pulmonica comes with a 30-day money-back guarantee, and is also guaranteed for one full year against manufacturing and material defects. The Pulmonica is hand-made in Germany by Seydel, the world's oldest harmonica manufacturer.

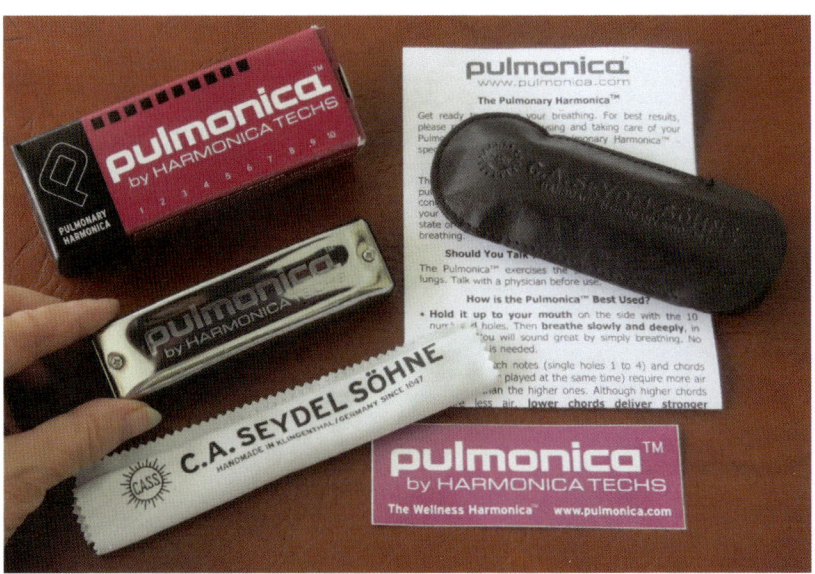

Play More, Breathe Better

The Pulmonica® Program

If you are under a physician's care for any lung disorder, check with that physician before adding the Pulmonica to your daily regimen.

Hold the Pulmonica up to your mouth on the side with the 10 numbered holes and place your lips over the cover plates.

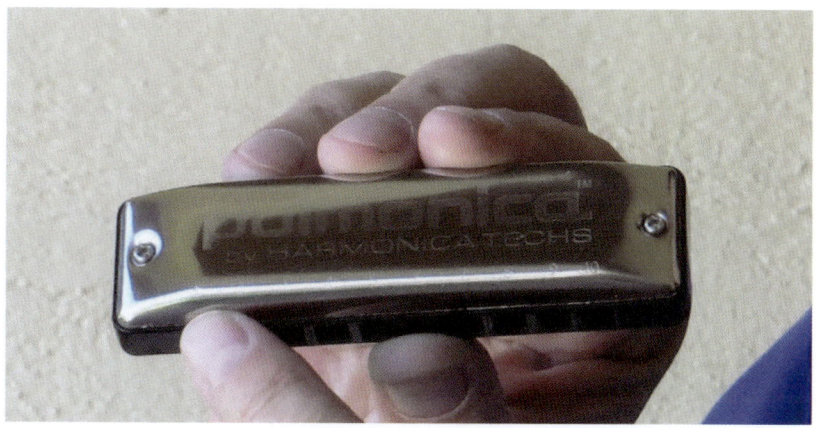

Then breathe slowly and deeply, in and out. You will sound great by simply breathing. No musical skill is needed. You are not playing the Pulmonica as much as you are using the Pulmonica.

Breathe deeply through the lowest numbered holes you can manage comfortably. Do this five minutes morning and night, and as often as desired for best results.

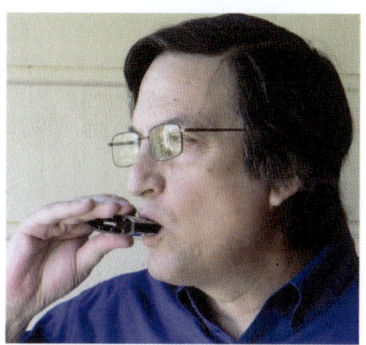

Meditating with the Pulmonica

By meditating or thinking only positive thoughts while you use the Pulmonica, you are increasing the benefits of relaxation and anxiety relief. Here are some examples:

- Close your eyes, relax, and maintain good posture. Try to concentrate on the soothing sounds you are making as you breathe through the Pulmonica and empty your mind. If thoughts enter your mind, view them with no more attachment than watching a flock of birds pass by.
- Some users compare the low notes to the ancient and mystical 'OM' sound and concentrate on that vibrational aspect.
- Imagine the Pulmonica's vibrations deeply entering your lungs and sinuses to loosen congestion. Try to feel your lungs clearing and getting stronger.
- Silently count the seconds you inhale and exhale. Exhale for longer than you inhale. Pause between each breath, both in and out. Gently increase your counts over time.
- Imagine the path your breath is taking, down your windpipe, into your lung tissues and pushing oxygen out into your bloodstream, nourishing all your body's functions. Then you exhale carbon dioxide that has built up and the process repeats. O2 in, CO2 out.
- Pray.
- Silently repeat "I Breathe in Love (pause), I Breathe out Peace (pause)", or just slowly repeat "Love (pause), Peace (pause)" as you breathe deeply from your diaphragm.
- Make up your own personal meditation mantra or use one of the many that Buddhist and other communities have used for centuries.
- Send positive intentions to loved ones, imagining them healthy and content.
- Imagine yourself healthy and content. What will you be able to do when you improve your breathing? Picnic in the park? Ride your

bike? Go dancing? Spend your five minutes twice a day visualizing your ideal life and be motivated to make it a reality.
- Ask yourself a question before you start using the Pulmonica, then let your mind explore it, or just wander for five minutes. The added oxygen might stir up some creative solutions.
- Read an inspiring passage and reflect on it for five minutes.
- Simply let the world go by while you just 'are'. Use your Pulmonica to help center and balance your mind.

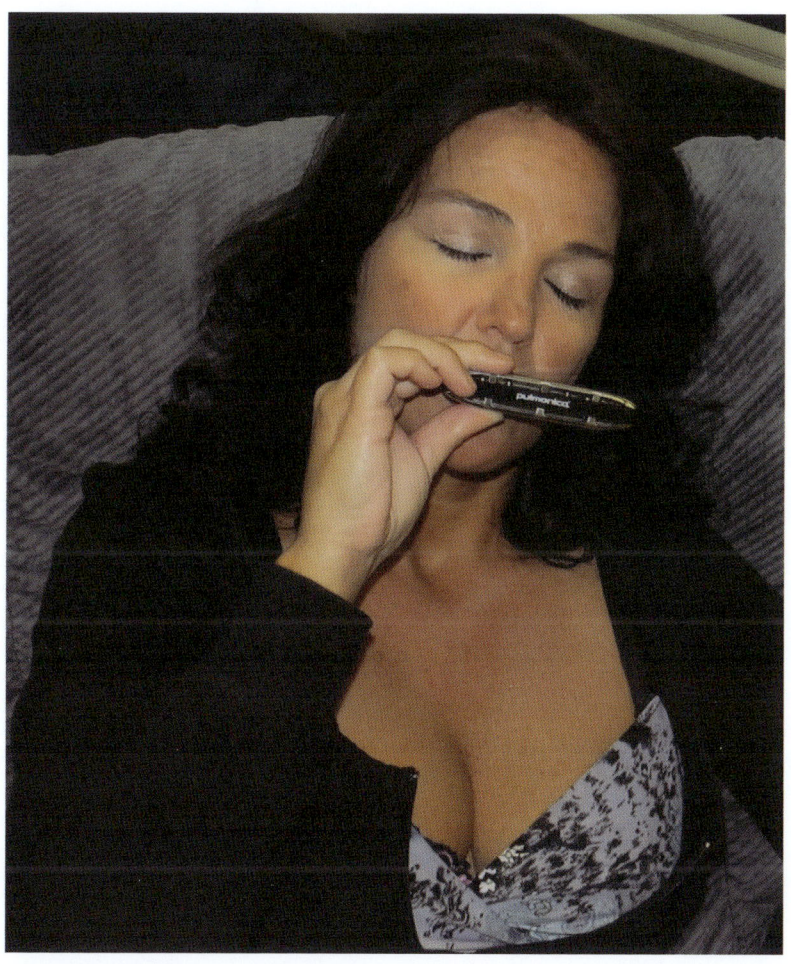

Surveys and testimonials show that the more you use the Pulmonica, the better you will breathe and feel.

People carry the Pulmonica with them and use it anywhere they can talk. The pleasing sounds are generally appreciated by those around you. Some people have reported being offered a tip.

The Pulmonica is also a great way to fill "wait time" during commercials.

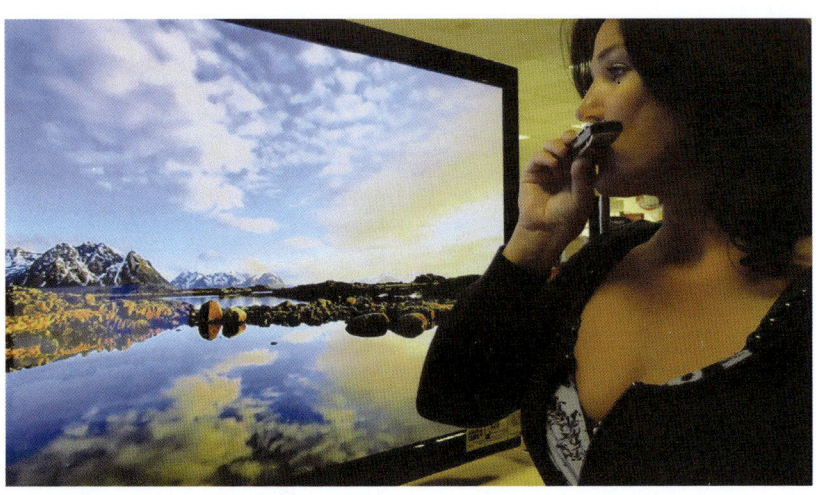

When there's waiting time at the computer ...

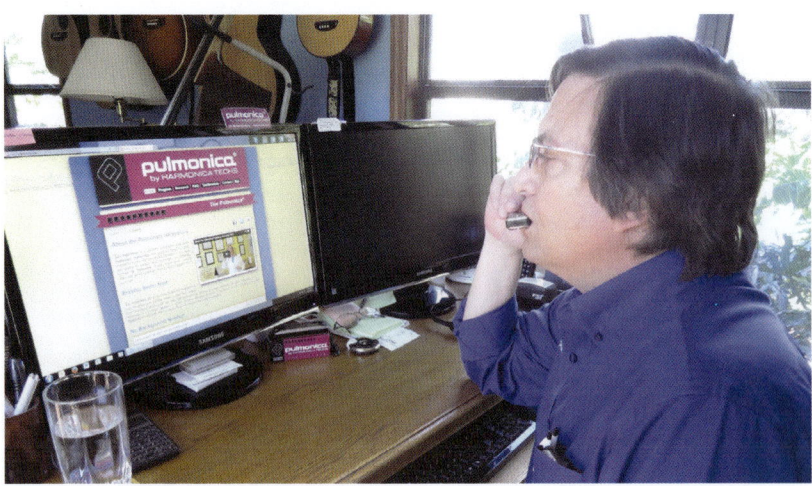

Or in a store....

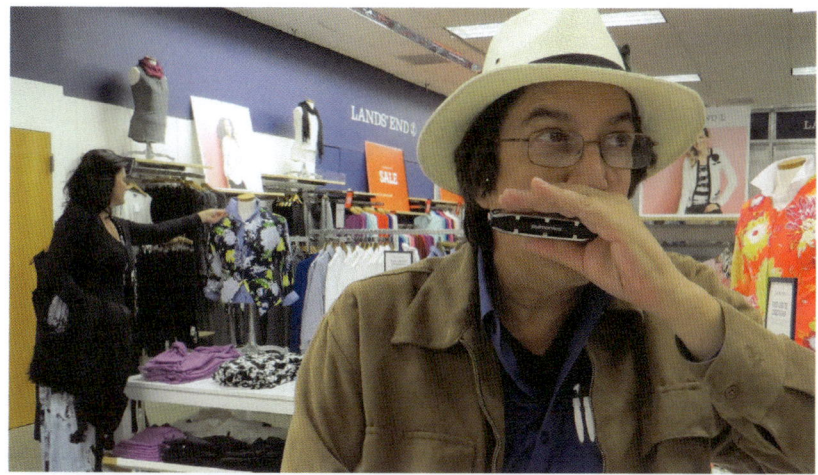

or any other time you need something to do while you're waiting. If anyone asks, tell them you're working on improving your lung health.

The lower pitch notes (single holes 1 to 4) and chords (multiple holes played at the same time) require more air and force than do the higher ones. Although higher pitch chords require less air, lower chords deliver stronger energy pulses to your lungs and sinuses.

Many people need to start by playing higher chords and work into playing lower chords over several weeks.

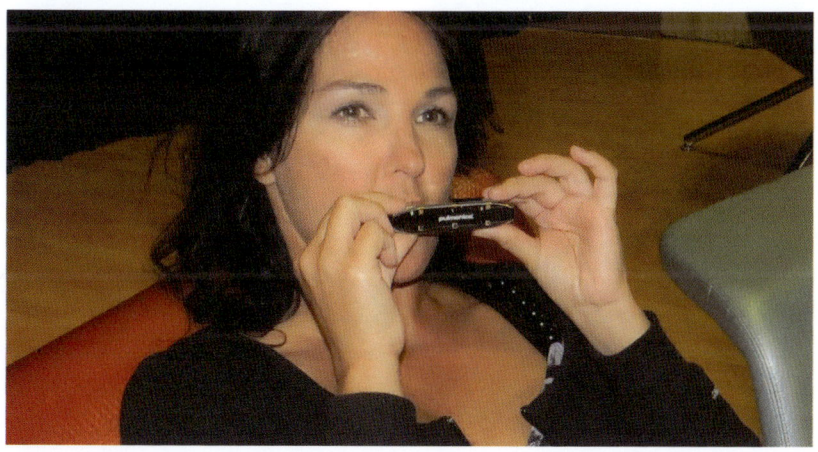

PULMONICA

Remember to breathe from your belly. Many people become shallow chest breathers and don't use the full potential of their lungs. Put your hand on your stomach and push it out when you inhale. Imagine your lungs filling with air from the bottom up. Your belly should move more than your chest. If you have trouble belly breathing, try lying down and repeat the exercise. This type of breathing is also called abdominal breathing or diaphragmatic breathing, and the method is an important component of respiratory therapy. Using the Pulmonica daily can help make belly breathing a beneficial habit.

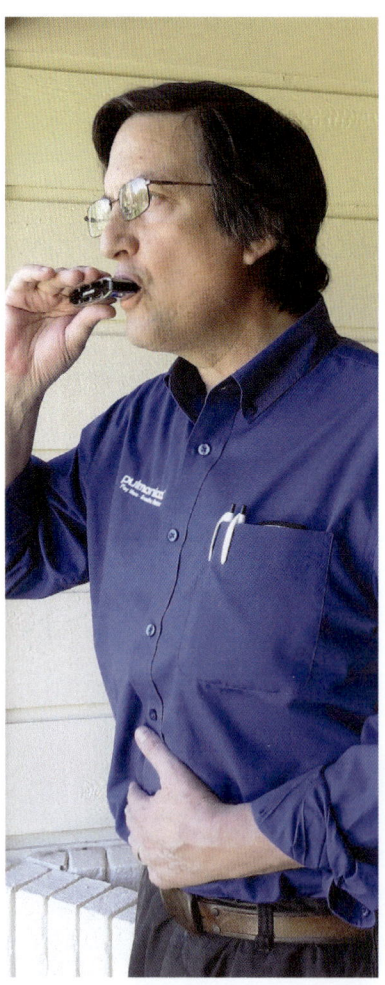
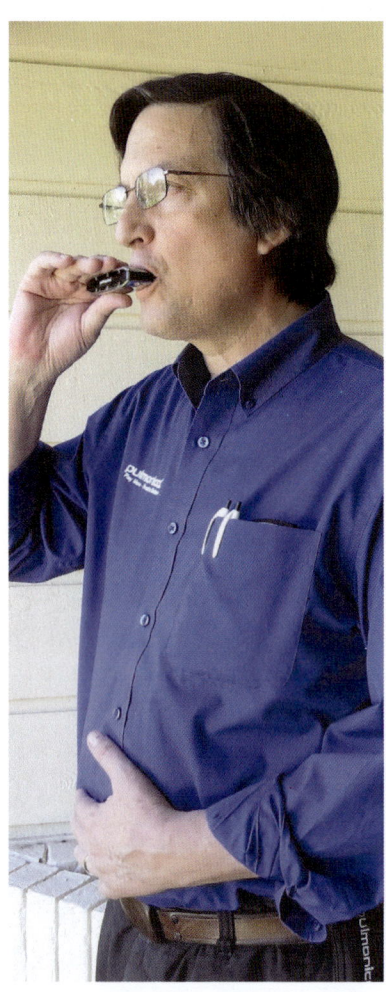

If your throat gets dry during use, drink some water and try inhaling through your nose and exhaling through the Pulmonica while you get used to it. When not using the Pulmonica, breathe through your nose to filter and moisten the air before it reaches your lungs.

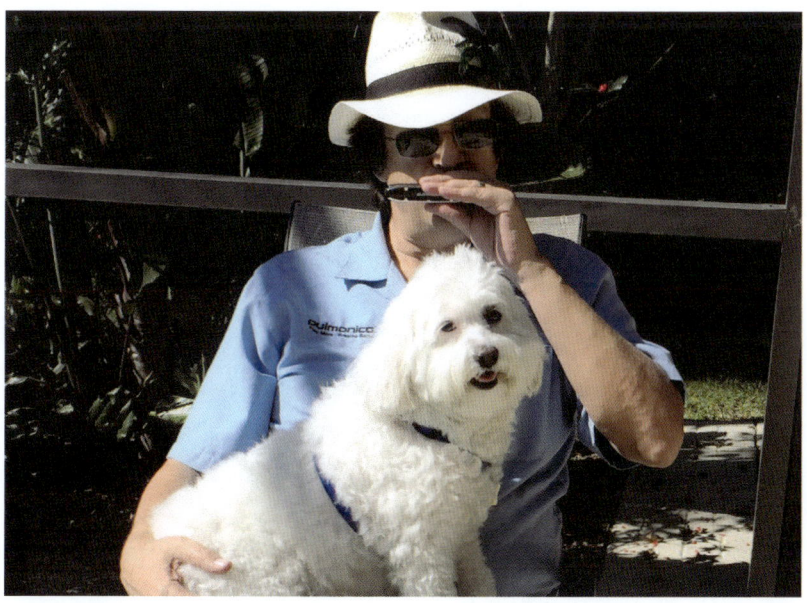

Play sitting down until you have experience. You might feel light-headed at first. If you feel light-headed, stop playing and remain seated until feeling normal.

When you inhale or exhale through a Pulmonica, don't use too much force. The Pulmonica has a built-in guide. If the reeds buzz on inhaling with low notes, you are breathing too hard.

Remember to use good posture and keep your neck and shoulders straight as you play.

Be aware of your environment when you play because you will be breathing deeply. For example, do not use a Pulmonica outside during pollen season if you are sensitive to pollen. Instead, play where air is clean, such as in air conditioning at home or in a mall.

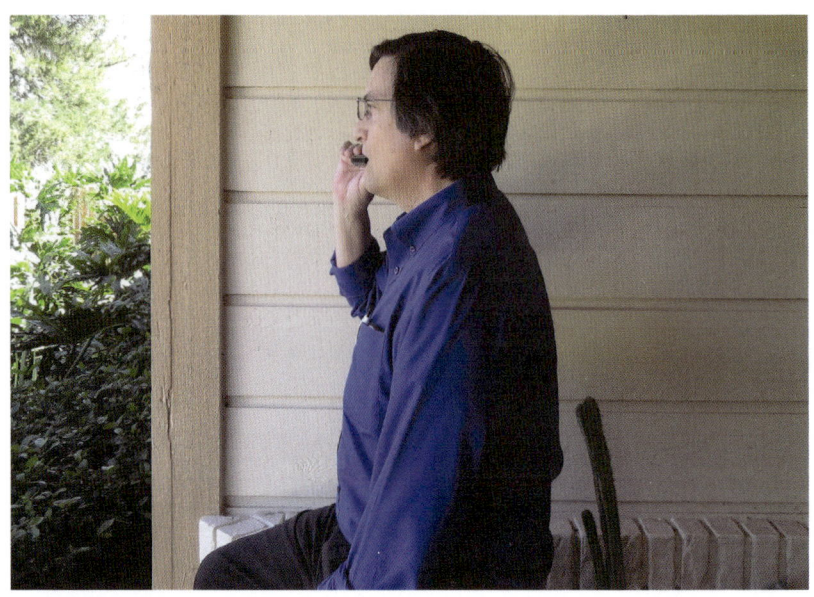

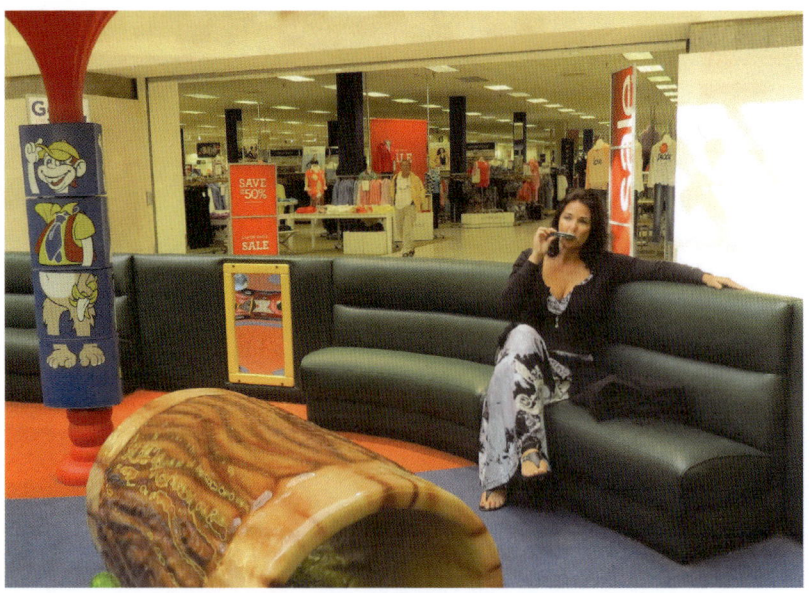

The Pulmonica is best used in combination with a pulmonary rehabilitation or support group, such as the American Lung Association's Better Breathers Clubs. Ask your physician for a referral, or look online for a local group. More information on what to expect in a pulmonary rehabilitation program is listed below.

To keep track of your breathing progress and changes in energy levels, make a note of how long you use the Pulmonica each day and how many seconds you can inhale and exhale. Additionally, a standard test for COPD that is used by lung doctors is how far a patient can walk in six minutes, so you might try that periodically. You can download our convenient Progress PDF from our website at **www. pulmonica.com** or keep a notebook.

Some people enjoy making sounds with the Pulmonica other than just breathing. Try chugging like a train and use the higher notes to make the whistle. You can also try saying the alphabet, counting to 100, singing a song, or whatever your imagination can think up. Remember to use long deep breaths for best results. Please send us a comment or video at Pulmonica.com if you come up with an interesting sound.

You can breathe in rhythm with your favorite music or a metronome. It doesn't matter if you're exact, the Pulmonica always sounds good.

If you want to try playing some simple tunes, download our MP3s and the sheet music and play along. Some people like to learn one song so they can impress their friends and family. There are a lot of free lessons online, just search for 'free harmonica lessons '. The Pulmonica is tuned to the key of 'G' for folk and country music. Learning to play songs is great brain exercise, but don't forget to use the Pulmonica with long, slow, deep breaths for at least five minutes twice a day to get the maximum benefits.

Pulmonica Care

- Do not share your Pulmonica.
- Have a clean mouth when using your Pulmonica to avoid food particles stopping reeds from properly functioning. Do not drink sugary fluids before or during playing, as sugary moisture attracts dust that can stick to the reeds.

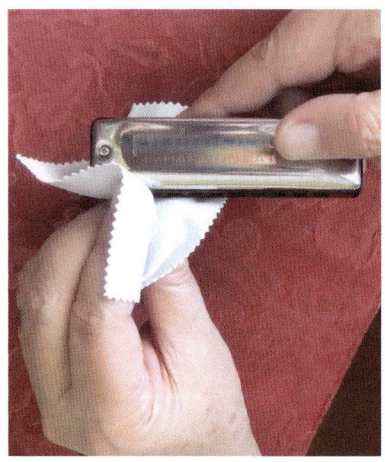
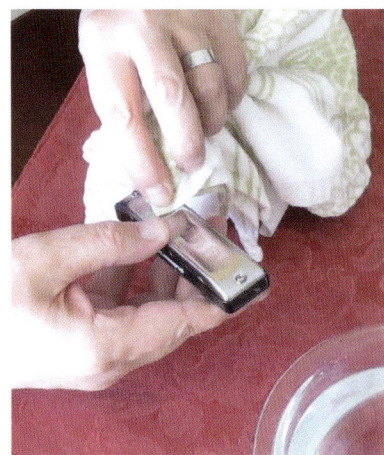
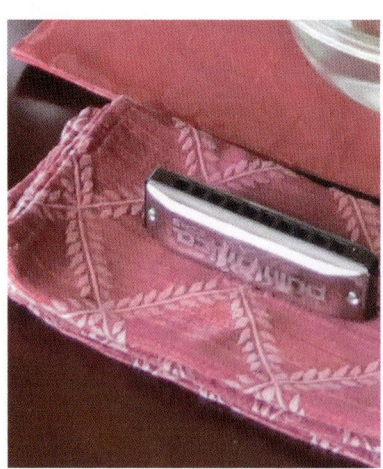
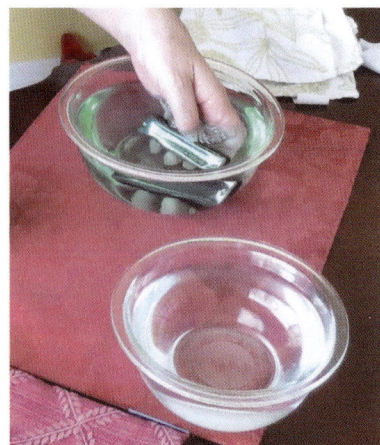

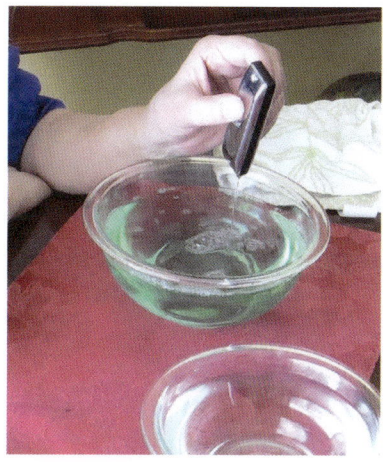 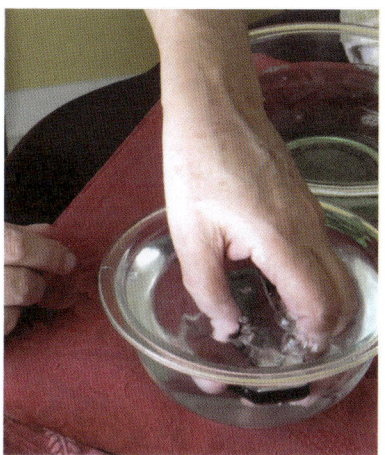
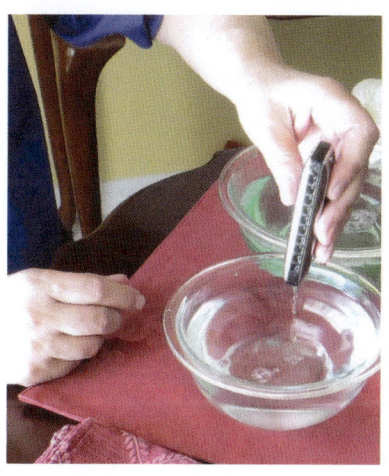 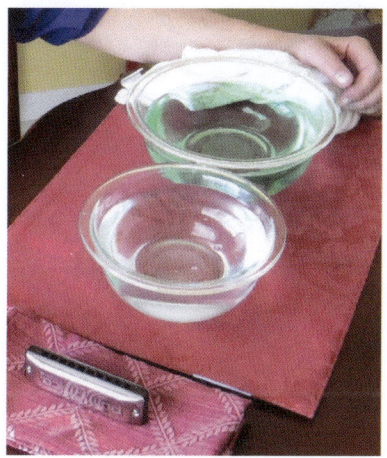

- Wipe the cover plates with the cleaning cloth after each use.
- Dampen a soft cloth with water to clean stainless steel covers as often as needed.
- Let your Pulmonica dry after each use before putting it away. Place it on a clean towel so that the numbered holes are facing upwards to drain and dry.
- To clean the inside, gently swish your Pulmonica in diluted mouthwash or plain water in a bowl followed by clean water, and let it dry thoroughly.

- Do not place your Pulmonica under running water or use electric hair dryers, as doing so can damage the reeds.
- Do not 'leg-slap' the Pulmonica to drain moisture. Due to the special weighted reeds required for proper function, this action can damage the reeds.
- Warm your Pulmonica to body temperature before using it to extend reed life.

Pulmonica Safety Information

- Safe for ages three (3) and older.
- Stay seated if dizzy from using a Pulmonica.
- Do not use if you have pneumothorax, advanced TB, lung pain, or are coughing up blood.
- Must be able to use without supplemental oxygen.

Pulmonary Rehabilitation Therapy Basics

Breathe deeply from your belly. If you're not sure if you're belly breathing, lie down with a hand on your stomach and breathe deeply through your nose. Your stomach should rise and fall. Keep practicing until this is natural all the time. Shallow breathing doesn't let enough oxygen get to your vital organs.

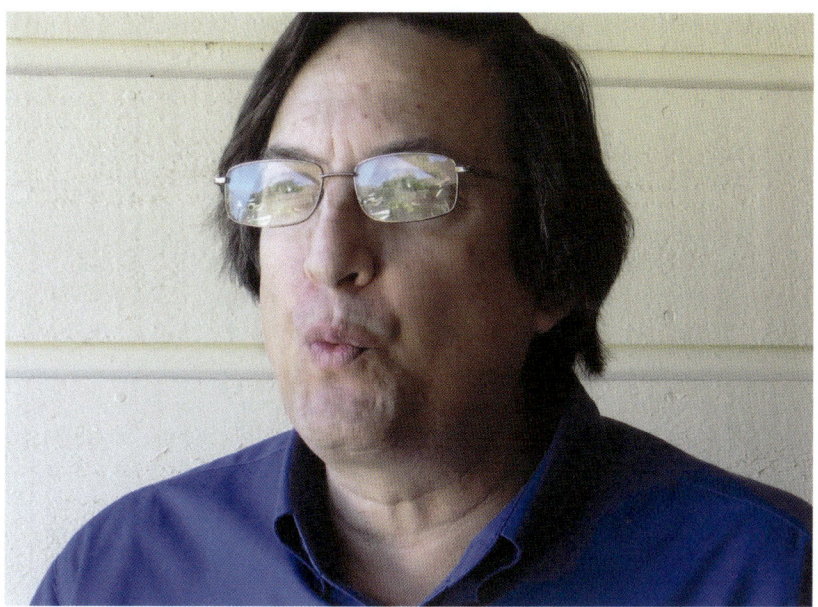

Pursing your lips when you exhale provides gentle resistance and strengthens your diaphragm. Using the Pulmonica daily will help make deep breathing a habit, providing gentle resistance and relaxing, meditative sounds.

Exercise as much as possible, again to get that oxygen and blood flowing. Try to do something active every day, and break a sweat four or five times a week. Lifting weights and staying strong now will help you stay independent later. The lungs are dependent on the diaphragm and chest muscles to work properly, so muscle strength is vital to lung function. Search online # for pulmonary rehabilitation exercises.

Pulmonary Rehabilitation Therapy Basics Continued

Take medications correctly as prescribed by your doctor.

Avoid triggers that can make pulmonary disorders worse such as: air pollution, cigarette smoke, very cold or very humid air, pollen, dust, animal dander and fragrances. You have a right to clean air, so politely tell people that smoke, perfumes, or animals make you sick. Even the residual scent and dander on people's clothes can be a trigger. Put a sign on your door so visitors are forewarned.

- Use good posture to keep airways open, especially while using nebulizer, inhaler, or Pulmonica.
- Get a flu vaccine every year and get a pneumonia vaccination every five years.
- Avoid sick people.
- Eat healthy foods in small quantities. Lose weight if necessary to make breathing easier. Smaller meals put less pressure on your diaphragm.
- Drink plenty of water. Staying hydrated will keep your secretions easier to cough up.
- Get enough sleep. Your body is under a lot of stress.
- Clear sputum with deep coughing, the huff and cough technique, or the Pulmonica. Examine sputum for changes in color or amount, and contact your doctor if you become sick.
- Find emotional support. It's tough having impaired lung function. Talk to a doctor or counselor about anxiety or depression, and join a support group such as the American Lung Association's Better Breathers Club.

Dear visitors

I have trouble breathing and it is made worse by exposure to certain triggers, such as strong scents, animal dander, cigarette smoke, pollen, and pollution. I do enjoy your visits, just please don't wear perfume or the sweater your animal likes to nuzzle, don't bring me scented candles or strong-smelling flowers, and don't smoke just before you come to visit me. If you want to bring me something, fresh fruit or _____ is always good.

How do harmonicas work?

The harmonica, also called a blues harp or mouth organ, is a free reed wind instrument enjoyed around the world. A harmonica is played by blowing or drawing air through one or more holes along a mouthpiece. Behind the holes are chambers containing at least one reed.

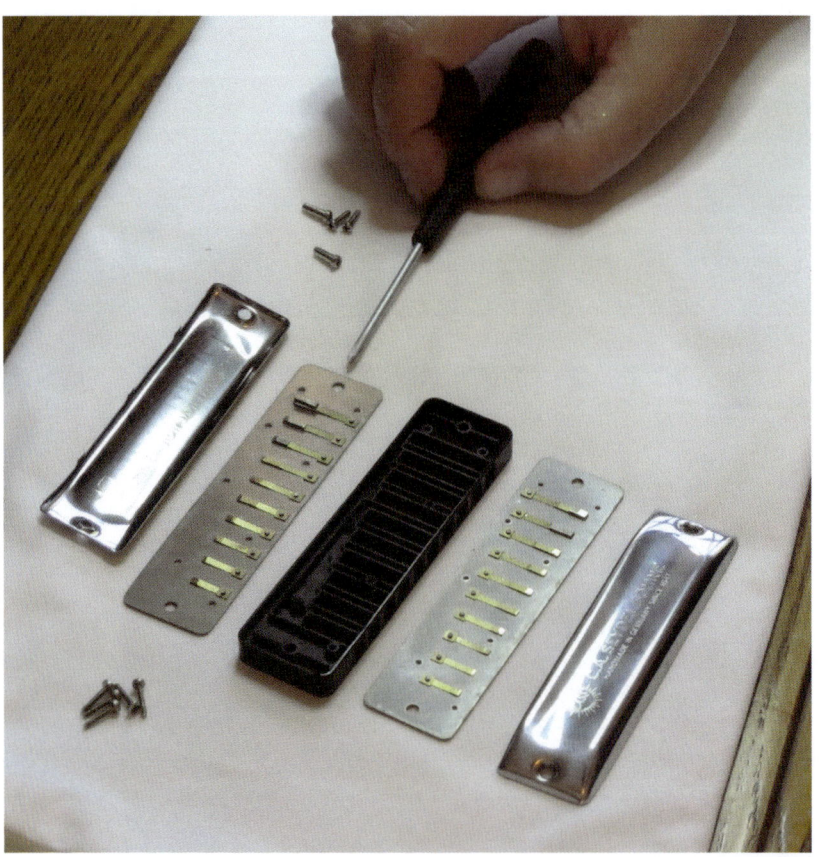

A harmonica reed is a flat elongated spring typically made of brass, bronze, or stainless steel, which is secured at one end over a slot that serves as an airway. When the free end is made to vibrate by blowing or drawing, it blocks and unblocks the airway to produce sound and a resistance that varies with pitch.

How is the Pulmonica different from regular harmonicas?

Most harmonicas have a few places that only sound good if you are a musician and know what you're doing. These discordant sounds are unpleasant to listen to and stop most nonmusicians from benefiting from this wonderful instrument. The Pulmonica is tuned to always sound soothing, with no tinny sound. The Pulmonica also has lower notes than most commercially available harmonicas, requiring specially weighted reeds that are hand welded on, and it is specially tuned to set up harmonics that vibrate your lungs and sinuses.

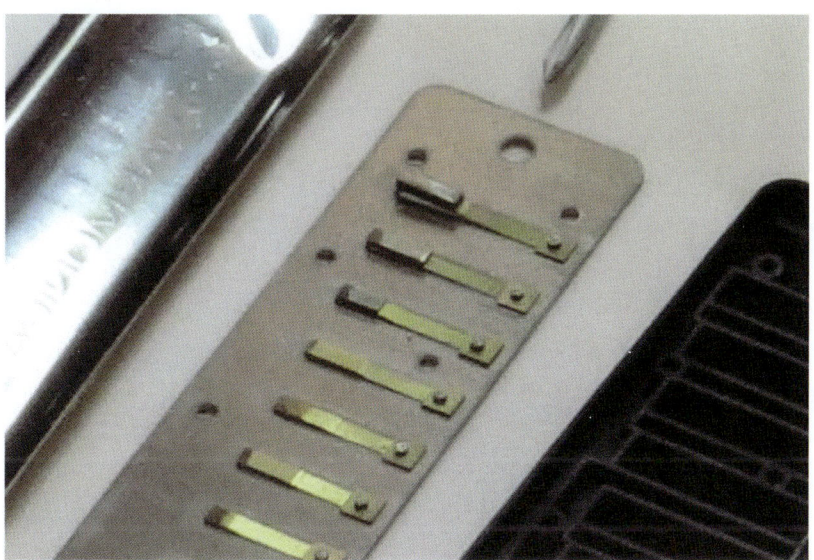

What quality materials are used in making the Pulmonica?

- Polished, stainless steel cover plates
- Recessed German Silver reed plates
- Machined brass reeds (20) for deep resonance
- ABS comb for rinsable design

Who makes the Pulmonica?

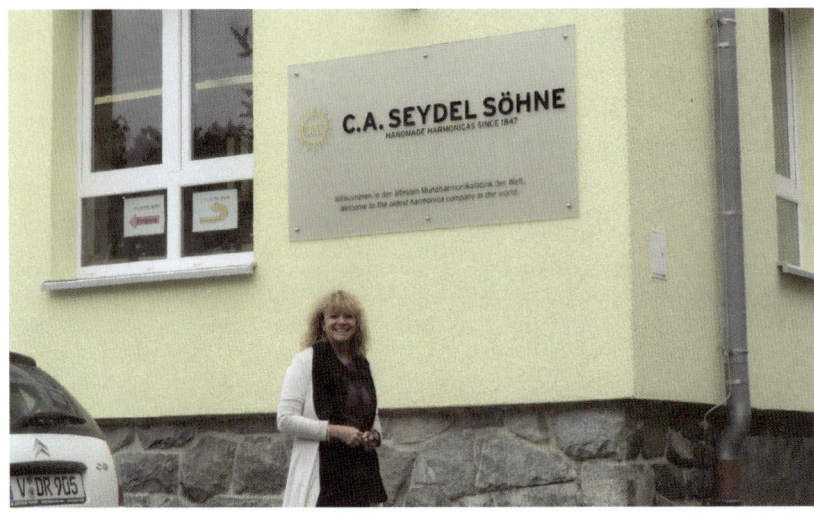

Our manufacturer, C.A. Seydel Söhne, is highly regarded internationally and has extensive global contacts. They have been hand-making harmonicas in Klingenthal, Germany since 1847, and continue to produce innovative products with the highest quality manufacturing available. You can find more Seydel harmonicas at www.Seydel1847.com.

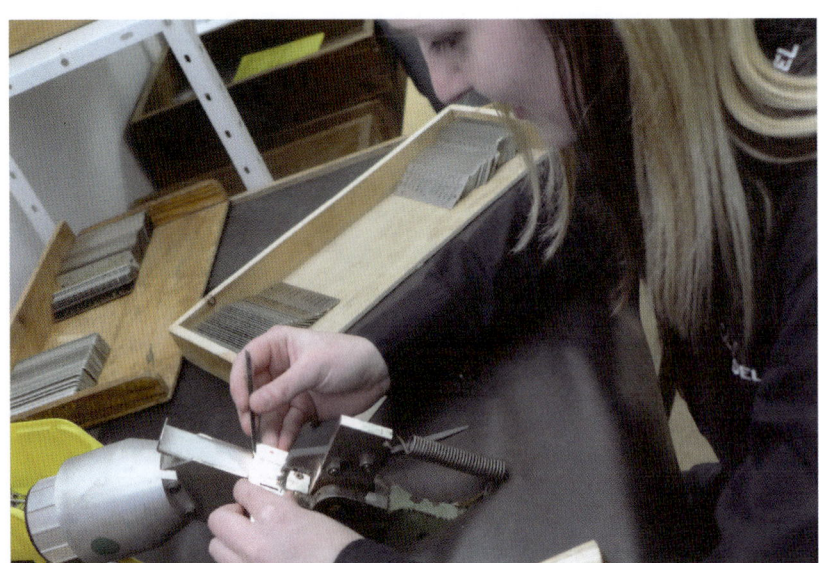

How does Pulmonica differ from other respiratory therapy devices?

The Pulmonica is the first fun, effective way to loosen secretions, increase the strength of the muscles surrounding the lungs, and gain the benefits of increased oxygenation and meditation. You're not just blowing through a tube, you're making melodious sounds that are pleasant and soothing with long, slow, deep, and complete breaths.

Why design a musical instrument for nonmusicians?

The Pulmonica is designed to obtain the benefits of deep breathing without the anxiety of trying to play an instrument. In the United States, only about 2-8% of people consider themselves musicians. That's a lot of people to exclude from the benefits of playing a wind instrument.

How was the Pulmonica developed?

When a family member confided he thought he might have emphysema, Dana Keller, PhD suggested he learn to play the harmonica and volunteered to try to play along with him. He soon learned that people lose significant lung capacity as they age and confirmed the health benefits from playing a harmonica. He found that commercial harmonicas were not tuned or constructed in a manner that optimized lung benefits, regardless of price. They were made for musicians. His wife, Mary Lou, wanted to benefit from this form of lung exercise, but she didn't want to learn to play songs on the harmonica. She just wanted to breathe long slow breaths against resistance, without musical intent. This brought a meditative and wellness aspect to the project. She also insisted that the instrument be smooth and comfortable to hold, so sharp corners wouldn't cause injury. By combining his knowledge of materials, manufacturing, and music with the determination to create an instrument anyone could sound good playing while benefiting their lungs, Dr. Keller developed the Pulmonica. And so, Harmonica Techs was formed and a medically supervised study was undertaken.

Why are you giving so many away?

For every twenty we sell, we give one away to a worthy charity, currently the Senior Friendship Centers health clinics in Sarasota, Florida. 80% of the world lives on $10 a day or less, and the working poor are more likely to be exposed to toxins and pollutants that can affect their lungs. We want as many people as possible to be able to benefit from this novel device.

What type of research do you sponsor?

We are interested in assessing the benefits of the Pulmonica in various populations. Our first study was with older adults who had Stage 3 COPD, but they were also part of a larger pulmonary support program. Ideally, we would provide the instruments for a study where the Pulmonica versus a traditional harmonica was the only variable. We would like to study the possible benefits to children with asthma and cystic fibrosis, as well as surgery and trauma patients.

Do you sell in quantity?

We retail on Amazon and have quantity discounts on 12 or more.

I would like to play some simple songs, how can I learn?

We have some sheet music and MP3s of simple, popular songs on our website, including: London Bridge, Twinkle, Twinkle Little Star, Oh Suzanna, America, and Auld Lang Syne. We have the Pulmonica alone, a guitar accompaniment, and the guitar and Pulmonica together, so you have your choice of how you would like to play.

For interested musicians, the Pulmonica is tuned to LLG, uses circular tuning, and produces the complete diatonic chord scale (G, Am, Bm, C, D, Em, F#dim) for over two octaves. The four-hole chords are G7, Am7, Bm7, C7, D7, Em7, F#half-dim. The Pulmonica can serve as a wonderful rhythm instrument in the Key of G. For soloists, it's a bit more challenging because the reeds, gaps, and profiles are set to optimize pulmonary usefulness, rather than musical playability.

If you would like to learn to play other songs, the Pulmonica is tuned to the key of G, and you can find backing tracks on the Internet to play along with. There are a lot of harmonica lessons online for people who want to learn to play a traditionally tuned harmonica.

We recommend the material from JP Allen at www.Harmonica.com. Many lessons are in the key of C. You can purchase harmonicas or arrange for lessons at your local music store or online.

You can find Seydel harmonicas at www.Seydel.com.

For a unique approach to playing harmonicas in medical therapy, visit Dr. John Schaman's website at www.HarmonicaMD.com.

How long should the Pulmonica really last?

That depends on how long and hard it is played, how clean you keep it, and your personal chemistry. According to the manufacturer, some hard players can wear out a harmonica in a few months, while harmonicas played only loud enough to make a full and pleasing sound can last for decades. That is why the force gauge is included. When you are inhaling on the low notes and chords hard enough to hear the Pulmonica buzz, you are inhaling too hard. Use easier breaths for both inhaling and exhaling. That way, the life of the reeds is extended as long as possible. When the Pulmonica changes how it sounds, it is time to consider a new one.

I bought a Pulmonica for my family member, friend, neighbor, patient, etc. Is it all right to share?

We highly recommend that you get your own Pulmonica so you can play along with them. Even if you don't have impaired lung function, the Pulmonica could benefit you by helping to increase your oxygenation. Some people tell us playing gives them energy, others say it helps them relax before bed. We would love to hear your story.

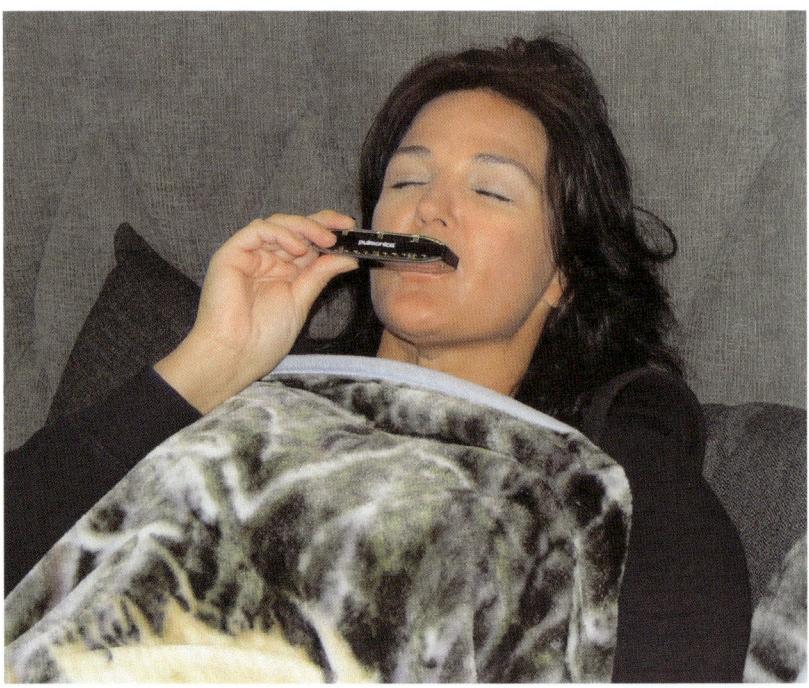

Something seems to be wrong with my Pulmonica. What should I do?

Contact us, please. You can send us a comment through the Contact page on our website # or call us at 888-382-9283. More than likely it's a clogged reed and simple to repair. We can walk you through it or advise you, but we do want to hear from you.

For Medical Professionals

13 reasons to recommend the Pulmonica to your patients:

1. Provides inhalation and exhalation therapy against progressive resistance. The lower notes are harder to play. Patients start around the middle and move lower as they progress.

2. Playing multiple notes together produces harmonics that vibrate the lungs and sinuses and help loosen secretions. Once the congestion is eliminated, patients can breathe easier.

3. Regular use promotes diaphragmatic breathing, which can then become habitual even without the device. This benefit alone makes the device worthwhile and useful for people with all stages of breathing problems.

4. The deep, resonant, meditative sounds are soothing and relaxing to the user, and pleasant for bystanders. This is especially important to someone who's worried about not being able to breathe.

5. Unlike traditional harmonicas, the Pulmonica has no sharp edges or tinny sounds, so it's safe and pleasant for people of all ages.

6. Handcrafted in Germany using stainless steel cover plates, brass reeds, and a high quality acrylic center, the Pulmonica is attractive and easy to clean.

7. No musical talent is required because the Pulmonica is tuned to always sound good. Just long, slow, deep, and complete breaths are all that's needed to get the benefit of this respiratory therapy device.

8. For those who want to try playing music, this device is one of the world's finest harmonicas and music is available on our website, www.Pulmonica.com.

9. With COPD readmissions being such a hot topic, having a new therapeutic device that patients enjoy using can only be a good thing.

10. Finally, a respiratory therapy device that is effective, empowering and pleasant to use.

11. Five minutes morning and night, and as often as desired throughout the day, and compliant patients should be breathing better in just a few days. And that should make everyone happier.

12. With a doctor's prescription, the device can be tax-deductible.

13. Now available on Amazon with a 30-day money-back guarantee. Quantity discounts are available.

Pulmonica® Research Results

From January through May 2013, a medically supervised study was conducted at the Senior Friendship Center in Sarasota, Florida, under the supervision of Dr. William Weiss, who has served as the pulmonologist at the Senior Friendship Center for 18 years. All study participants were tested for and had Stage 3 COPD (chronic obstructive pulmonary disease) without other serious comorbidity, such as CHF (congestive heart failure).

Nine COPD patients completed the pulmonary rehabilitation study, which included intake and exit interviews, spirometry, six minute walk and quality of life assessments, educational programs on proper breathing techniques and use of medications, a brief exercise program using stretching, hand weights and chair exercises, and use of a novel harmonic device, the Pulmonica Pulmonary Harmonica. This device requires no musical talent, and participants were encouraged to simply breathe long, slow deep breaths in and out through the lowest holes they could manage comfortably. The lower holes provide a deep resonant sound that vibrates through the lungs and sinuses and is pleasant and meditative.

Results from the Medically Supervised Trial were extremely positive. All of the patients improved in their quality of life assessment, spirometry, six minute walk, and everyone agreed that the more they played the Pulmonica, the better they breathed and felt.

Quantitative Results

The quantitative results are shown in Table 1. The table shows the measure, baseline result, absolute change, p-value, upper and lower 95% confidence intervals, and relative change. All gathered data were used for the statistical results. Although the study was small in size, with more studies to come, the p-values statistics account for size.

Measure (N=9)	Baseline Average	8 Weeks Later*	Relative Change
Quality of Life Survey	90	101	+13%
6-Minute Walk, feet	383	447	+17%
FEV1	40%	54%	+34%
FVC	42%	61%	+46%
* All increases statistically significant at the $p < .05$ level.			

Graphically, the results are shown in Figure 1.

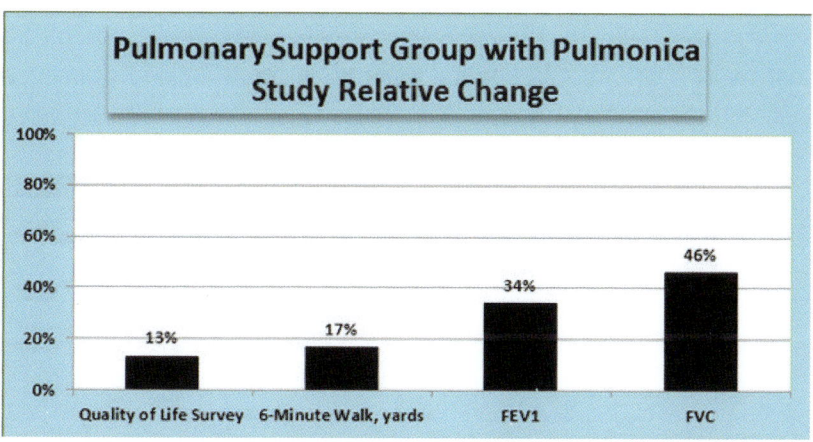

Relative Change

Clearly, participants benefited sufficiently from the overall program that included clinical education, mild exercise, and use of the Pulmonica to warrant more detailed study and analysis. If you are a researcher interested in conducting research on the Pulmonica Pulmonary Harmonica, please leave a comment on our website and we will contact you.

Qualitative Findings

The following qualitative findings were unanimous across study participants and are highly significant ($p < .001$).

The more people played the Pulmonica – the better they could breathe

The more people played the Pulmonica – the clearer their lungs were

The more people played the Pulmonica – the more energy they had

The more people played the Pulmonica – the better they felt

Testimonials included

Loosened fluids in lungs and sinuses, allowing people to cough up secretions and breathe easier

Decreased rescue inhaler and nebulizer use

Decreased auxiliary oxygen use

Feeling calmer because of the meditative aspect of playing

Better sleep

Walking further

Singing better

Stronger talking voice

Getting out again, such as to the beach and shopping

Doing housework for themselves again

Standing and walking without need of supports, such as walkers or canes

Happier

Joining a gym and riding a bike

More hopeful about their future

More studies are in process investigating the Pulmonica in home health care, as a smoking cessation aide, and in a hospital setting. Research inquiries are welcome at dana@pulmonica.com.

Printed in Great Britain
by Amazon